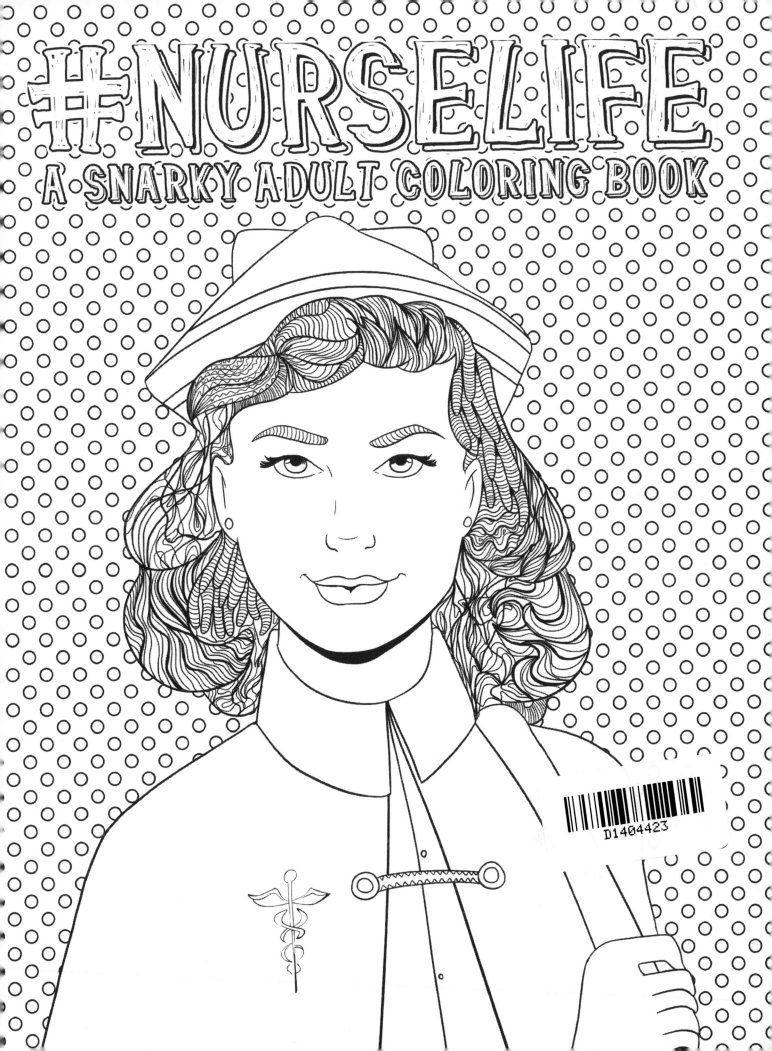

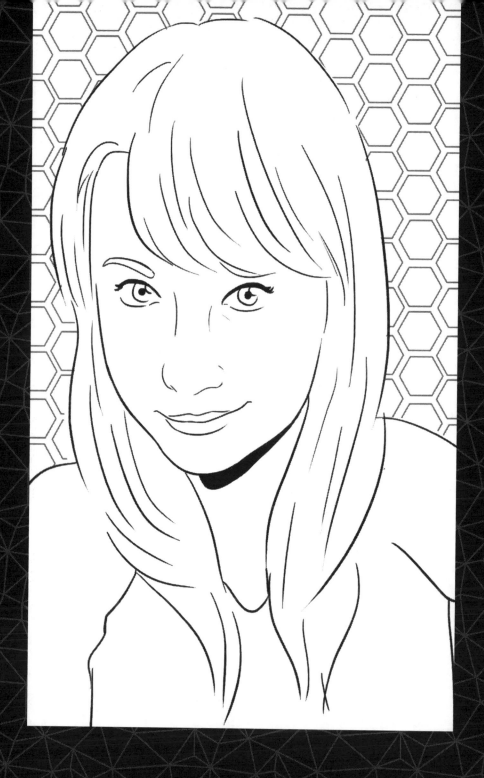

Illustrated by Micaela

ISBN-13: 978-1533081964
ISBN-10: 1533081964

#NURSELIFE

Nurses, you truly are angels in disguise. In the most trying times and stressful circumstances, you are compassionate, kind, wise, and patient beyond measure. But let's be real. All that self-sacrifice must give you daydreams of hijacking some gurneys and pushing each other straight to Mexico for vacation. Well, put back the gurneys and pick up this Coloring Book instead! With each page you color, feel the exhaustion and stress melt away like so many ocean waves and margaritas.

Papeterie Bleu

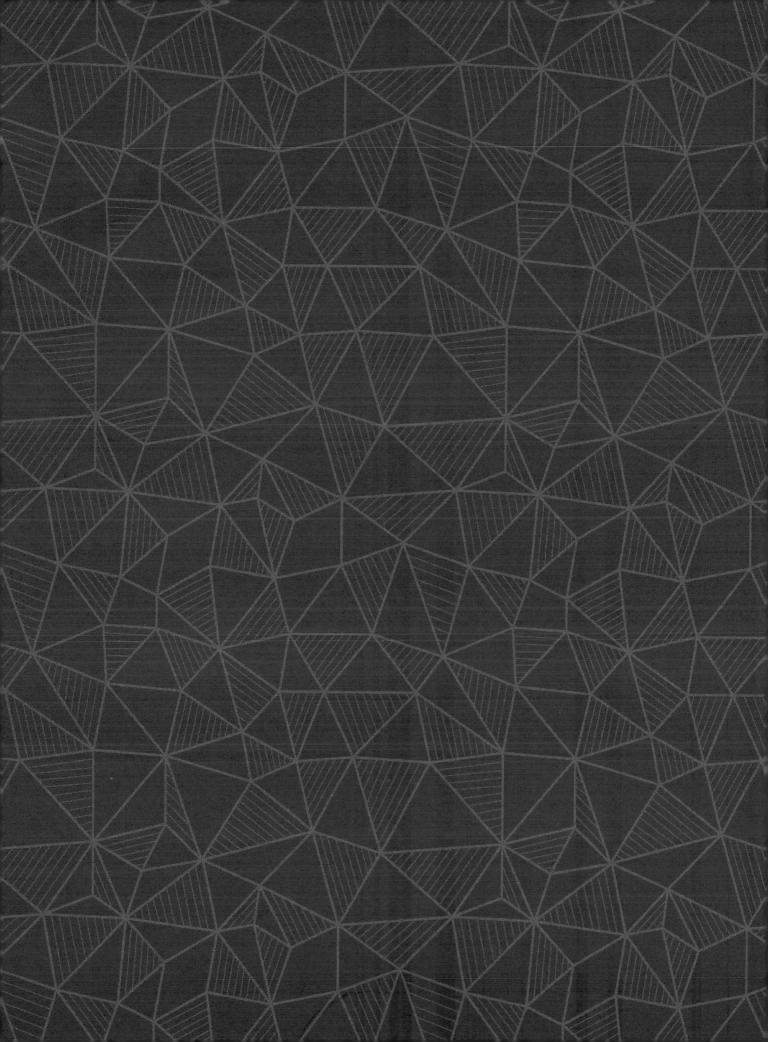

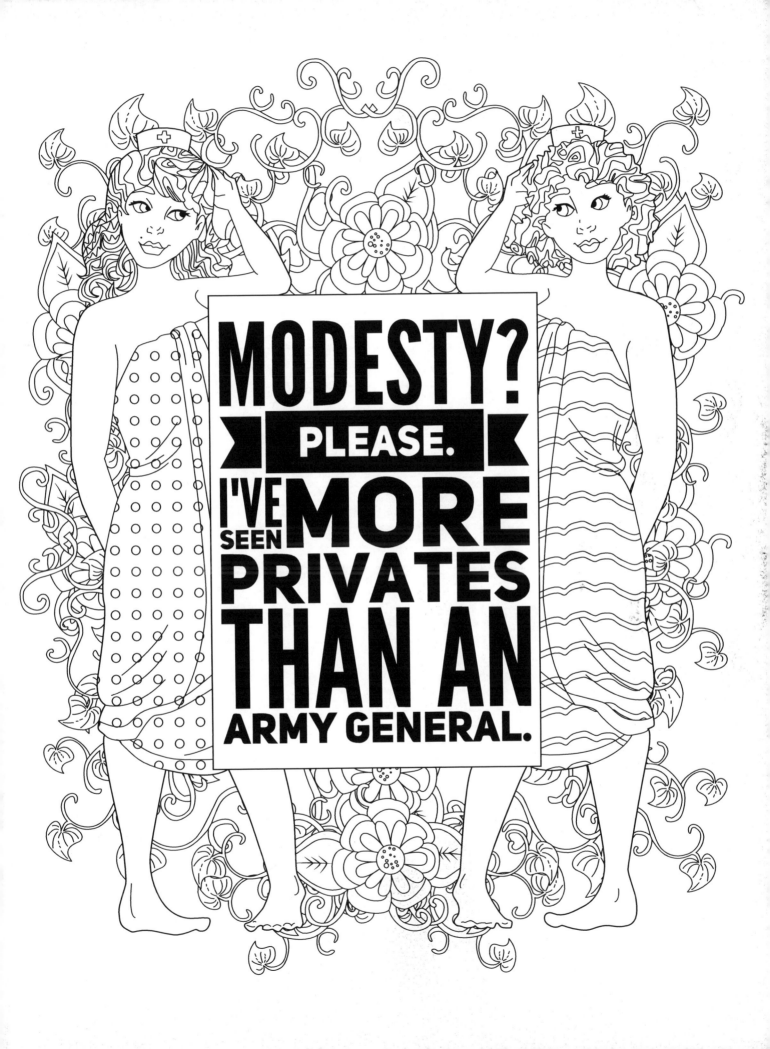

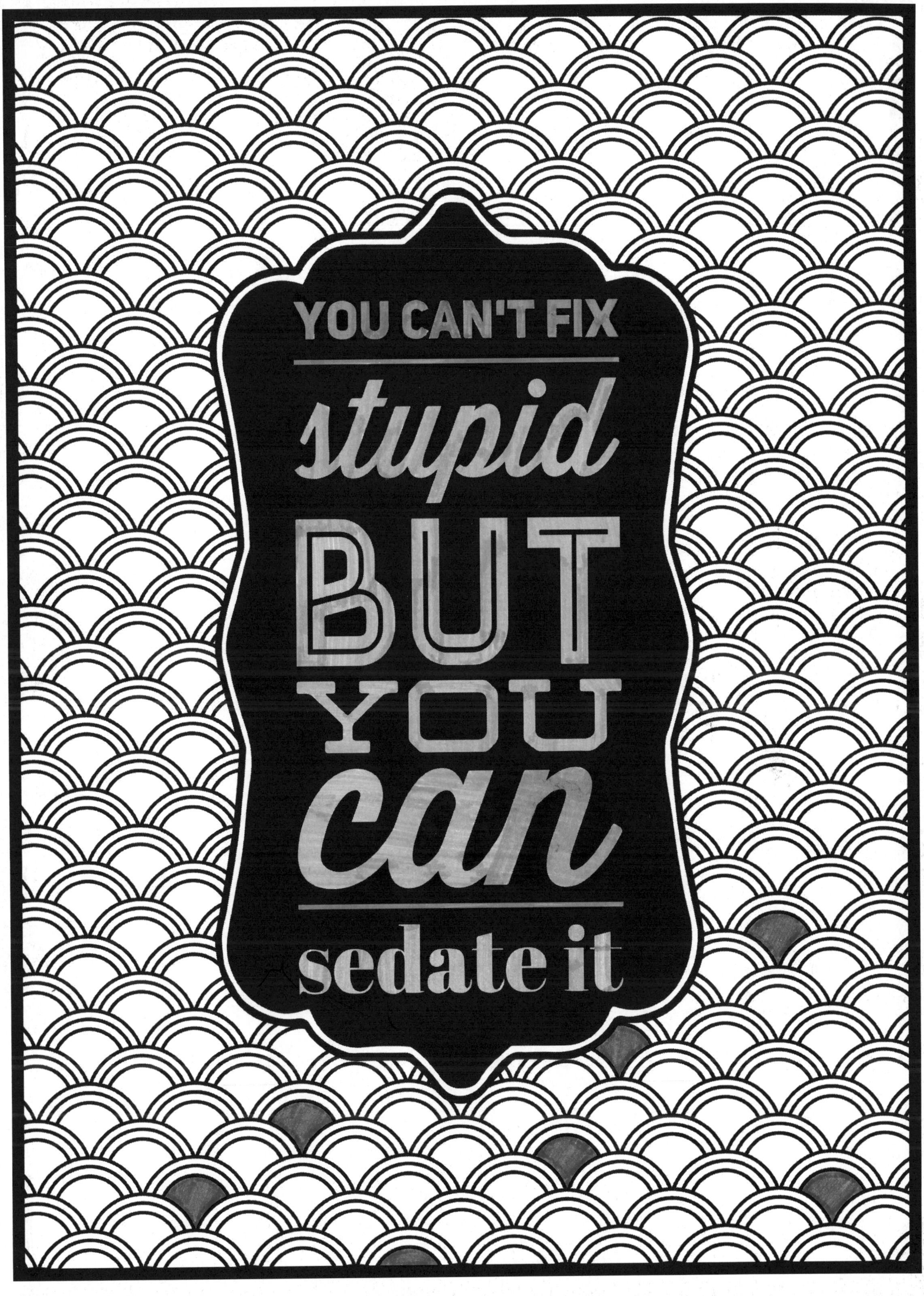
YOU CAN'T FIX
stupid
BUT
YOU
can
sedate it

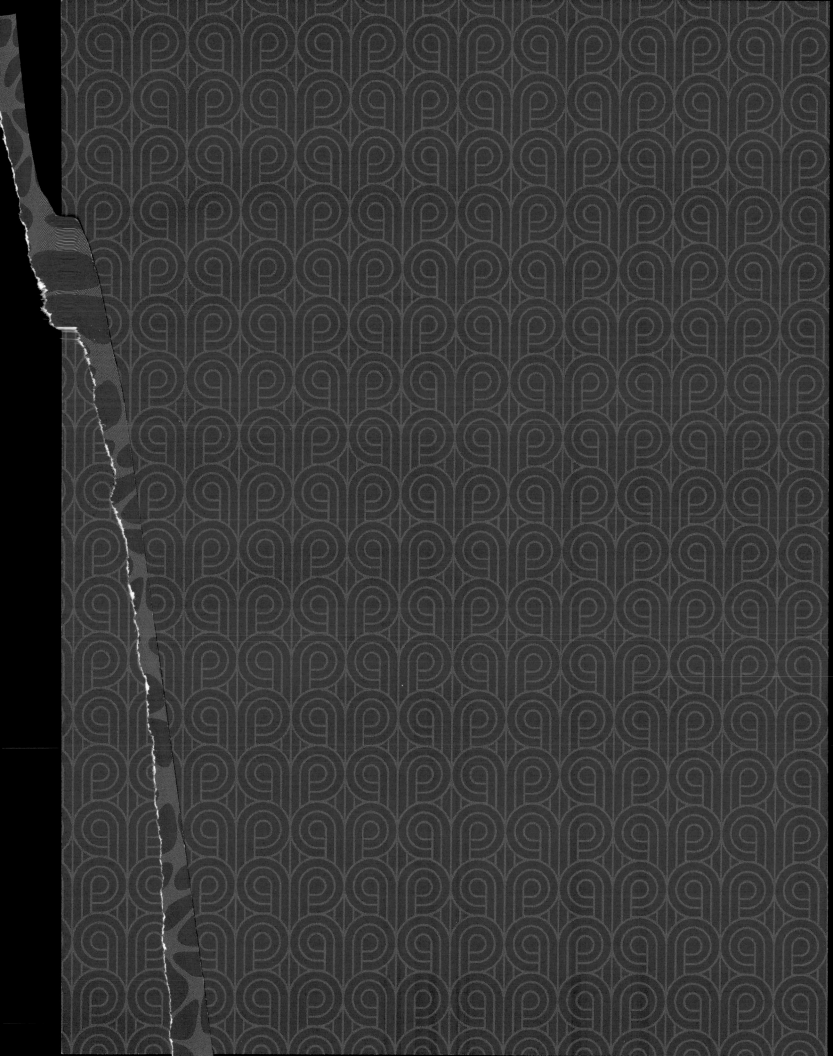

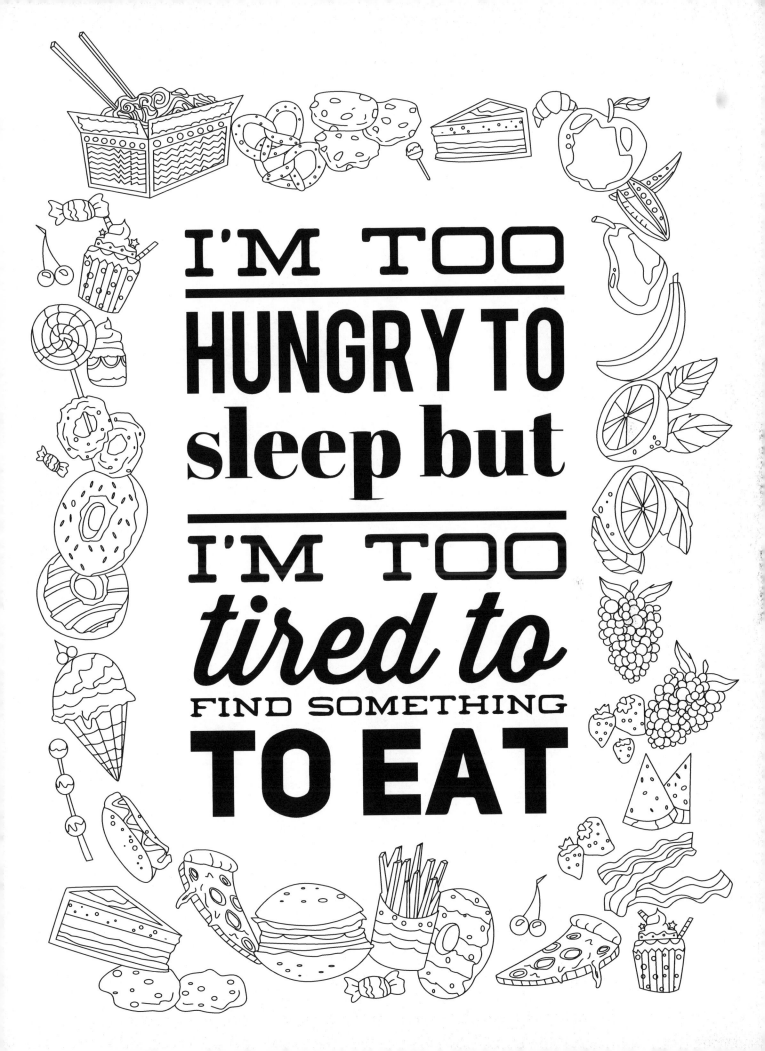

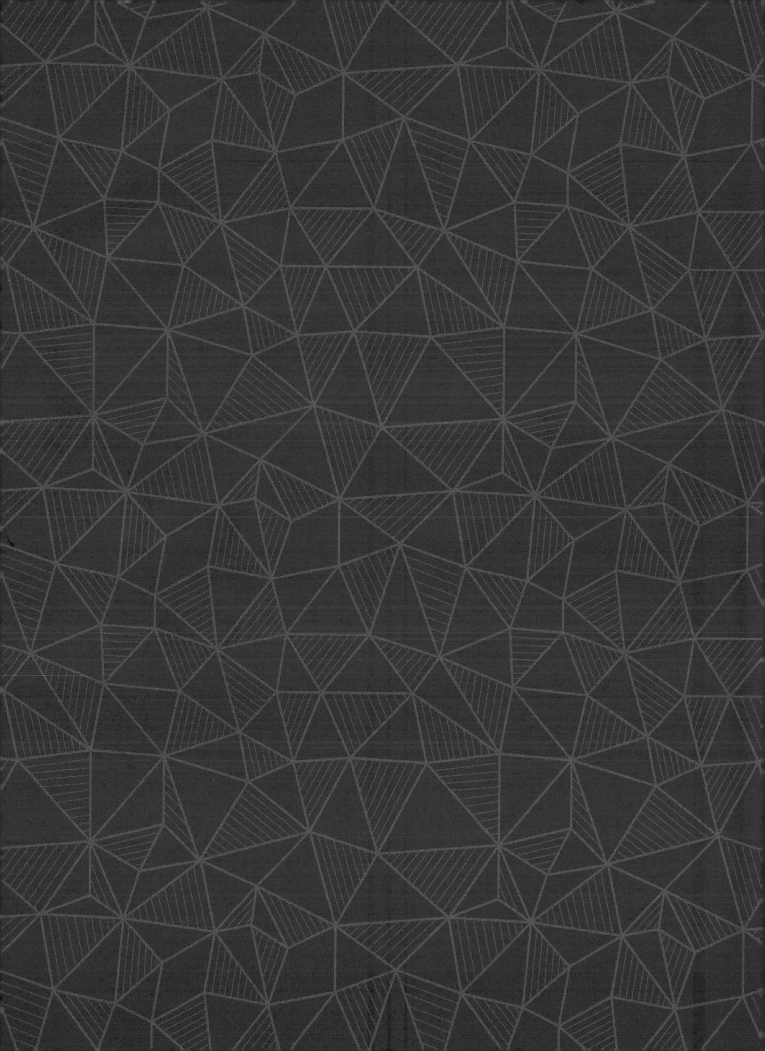

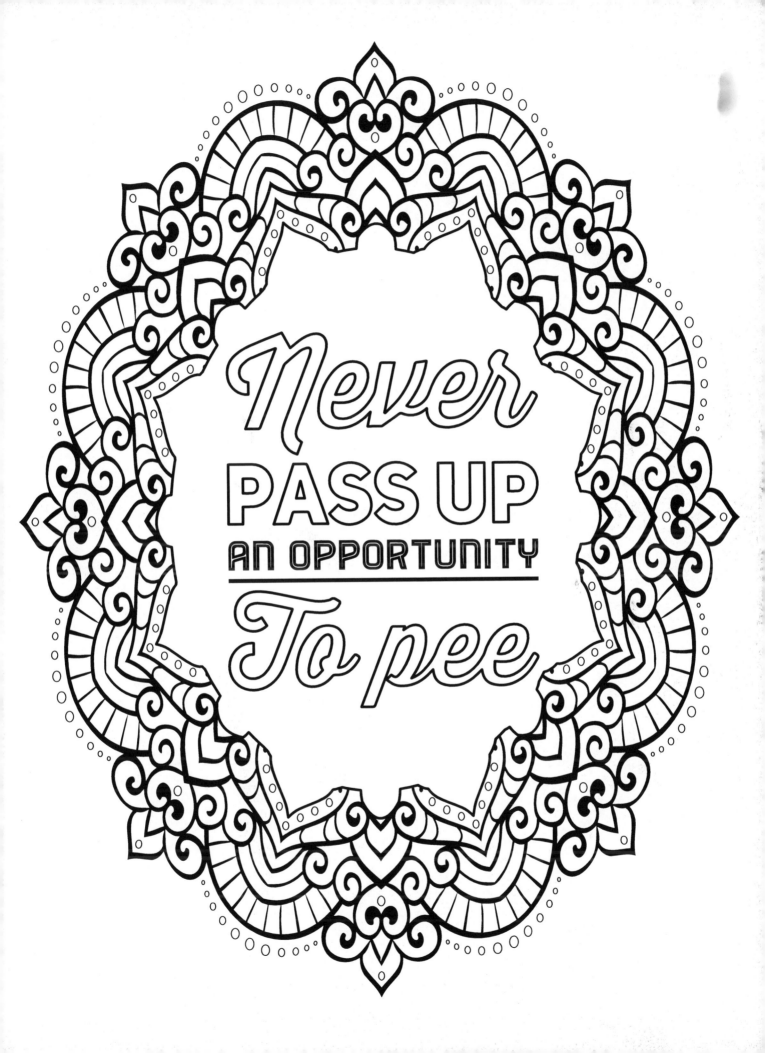

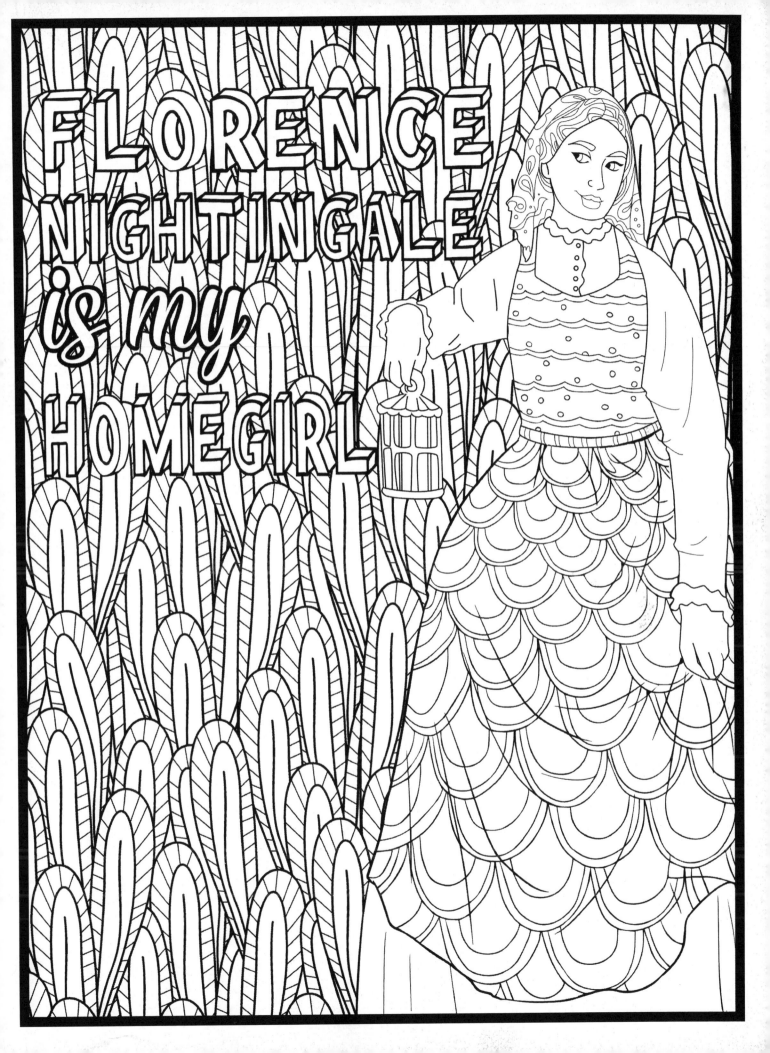

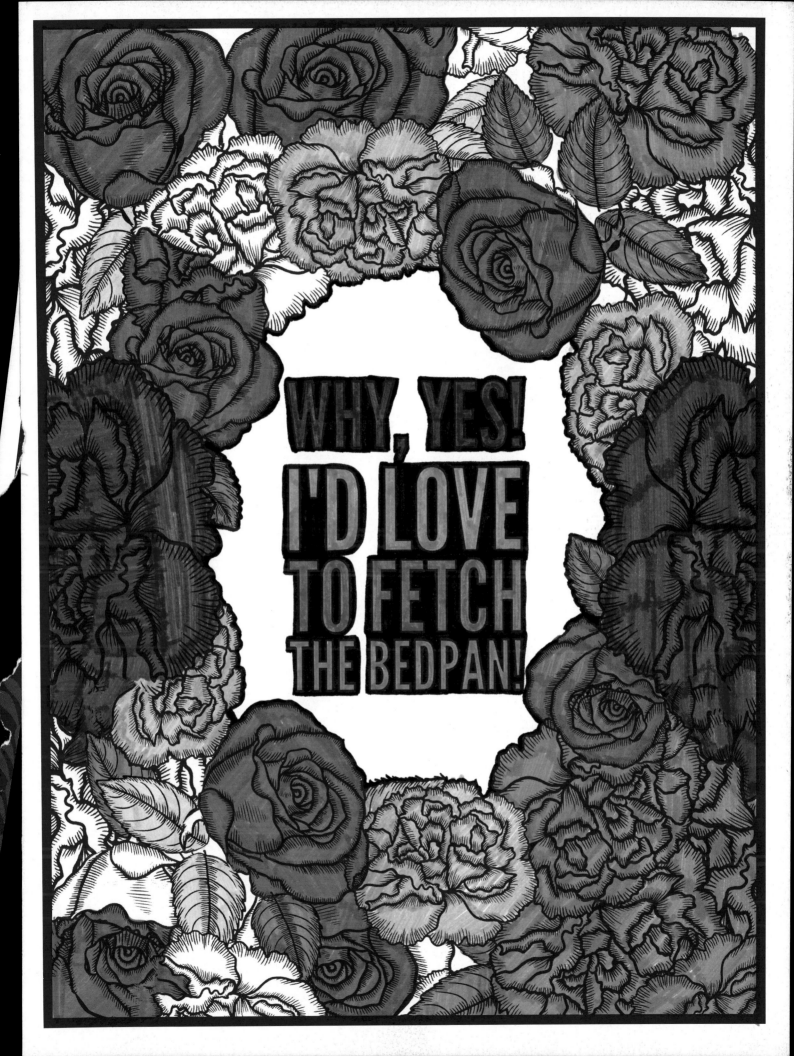

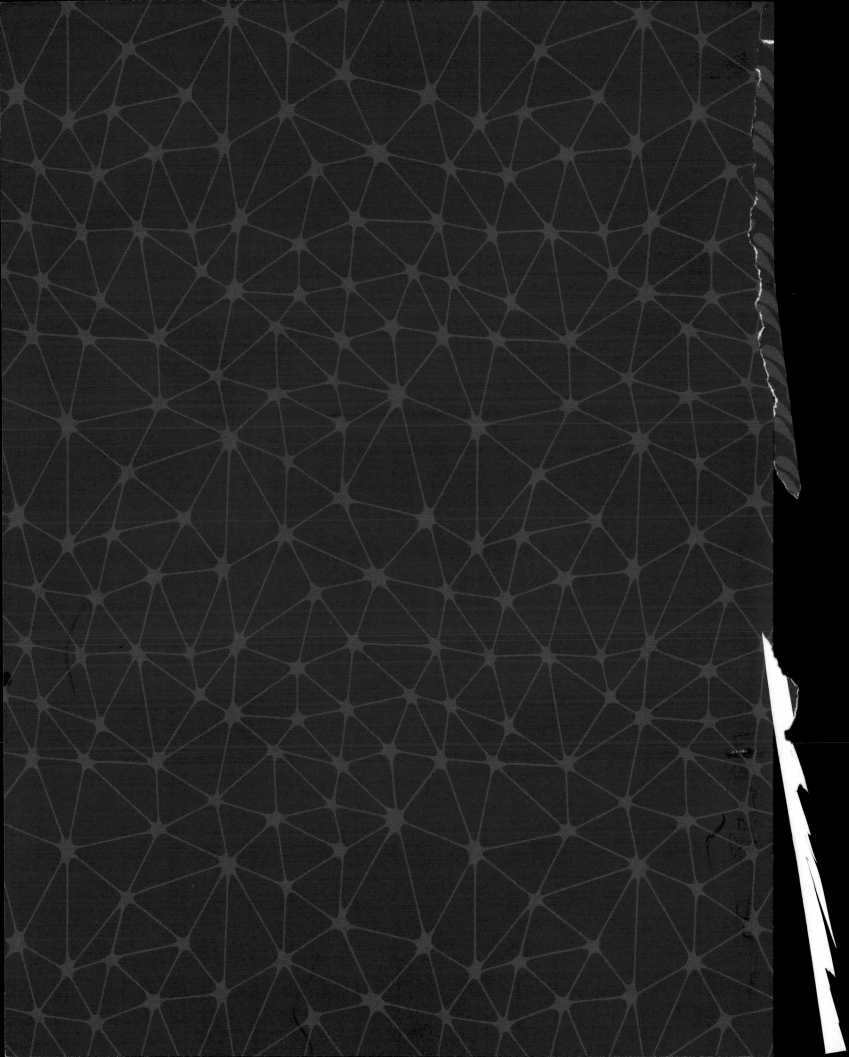

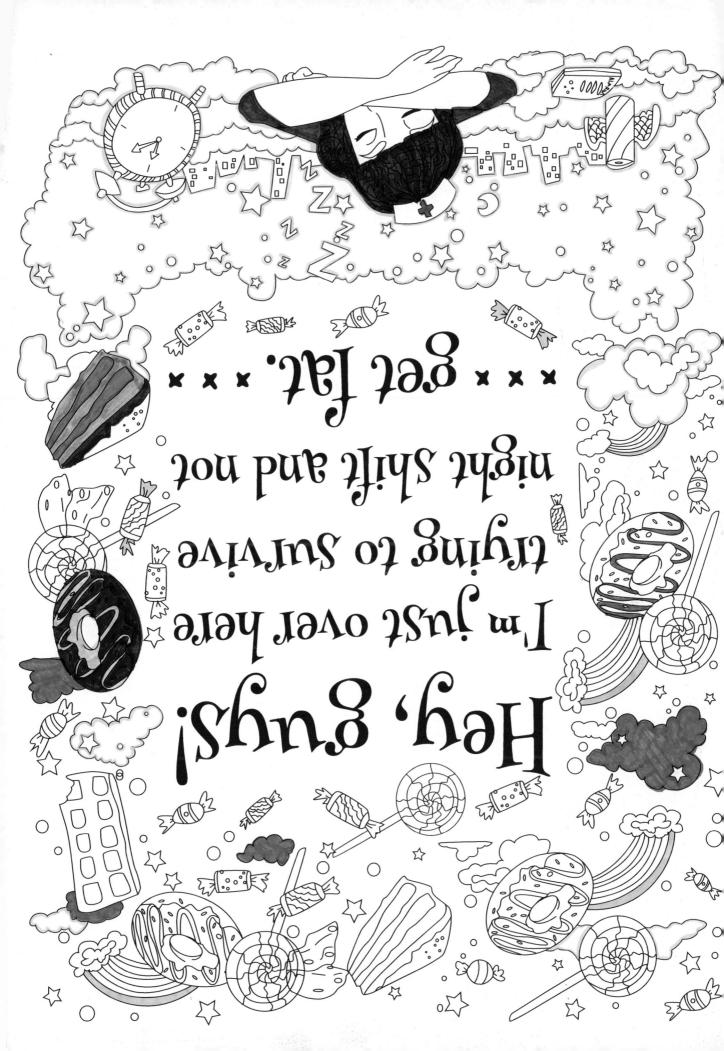

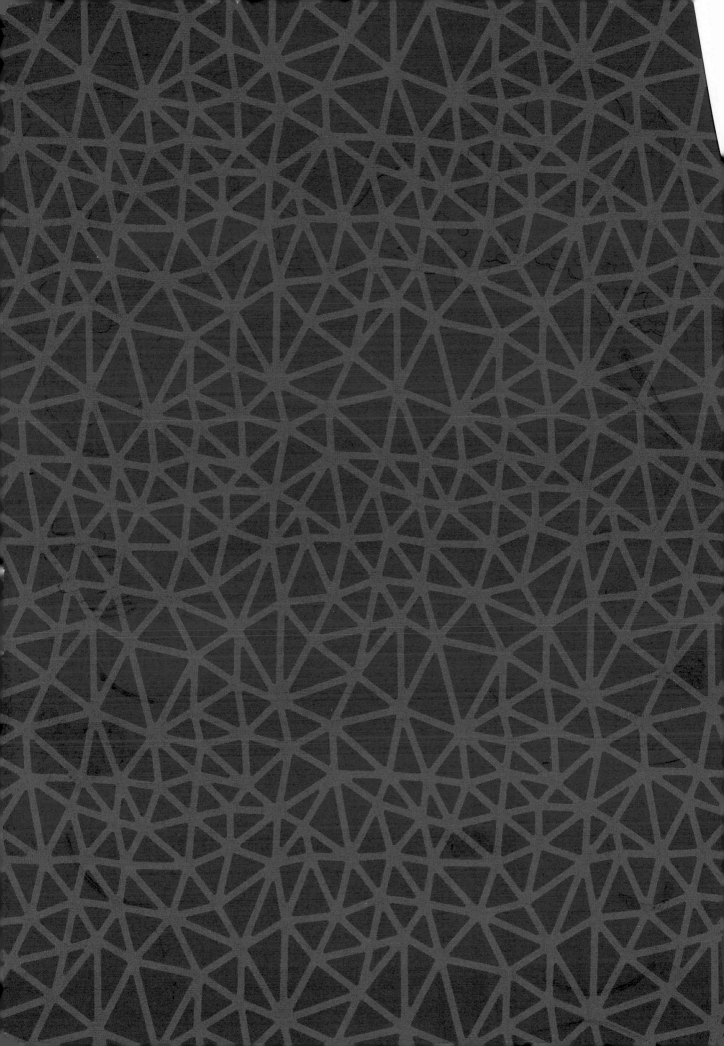

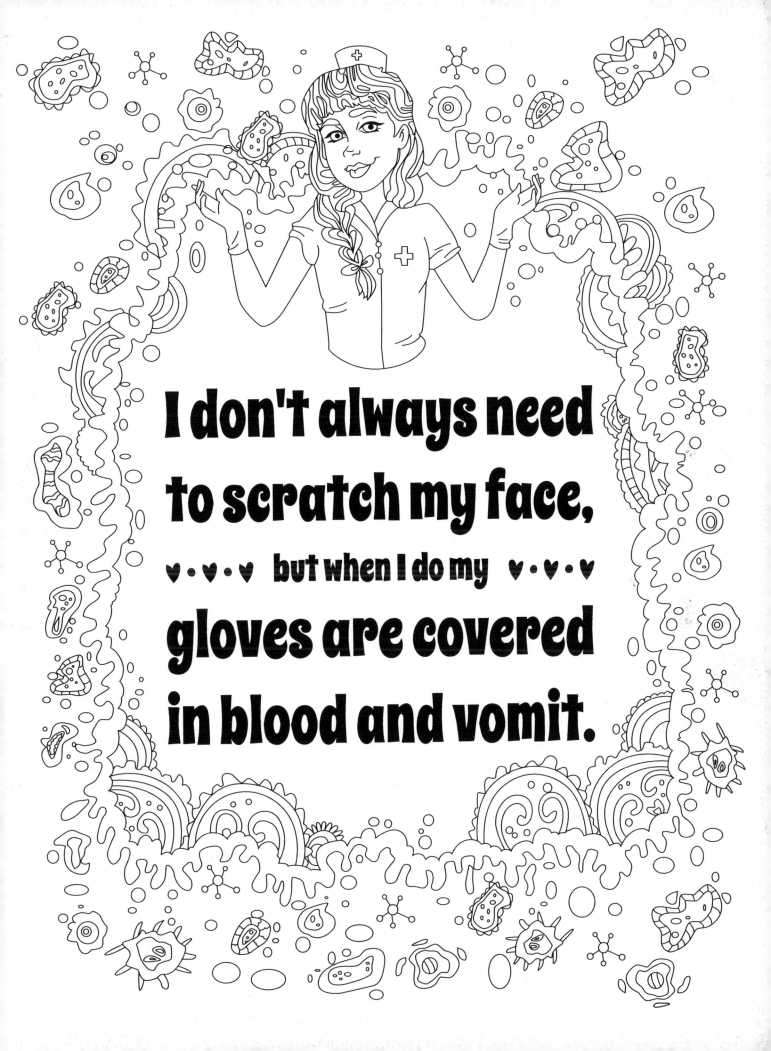

I don't always need to scratch my face, ♥ • • ♥ but when I do my ♥ • • ♥ gloves are covered in blood and vomit.

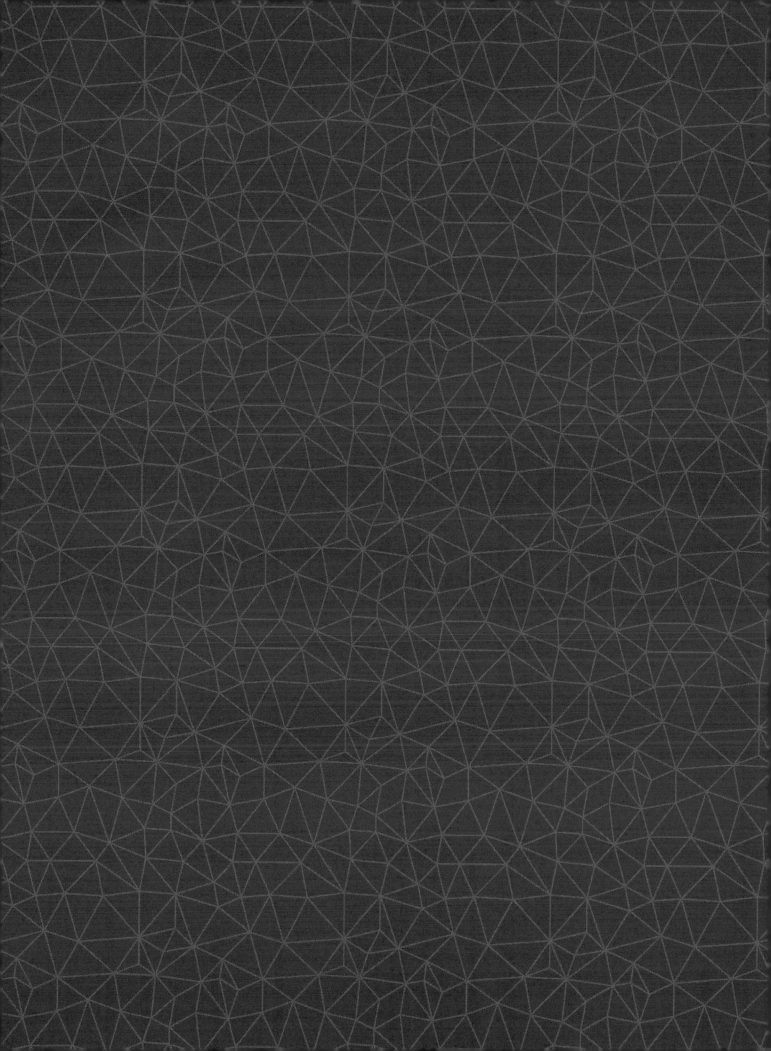

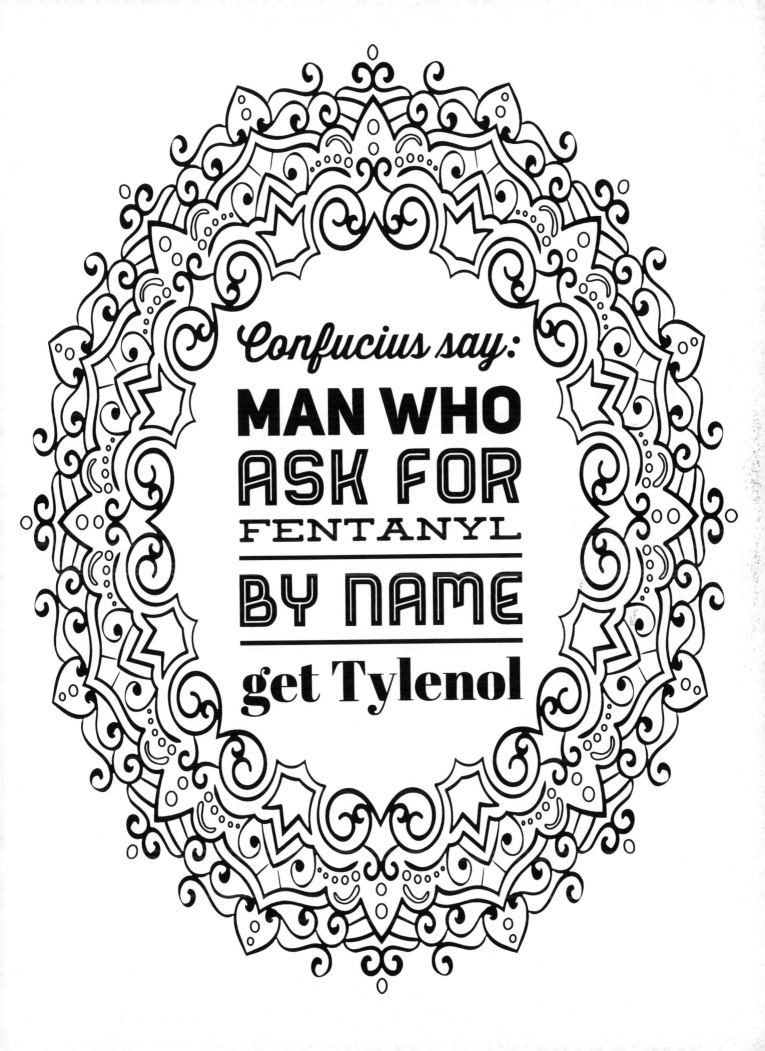

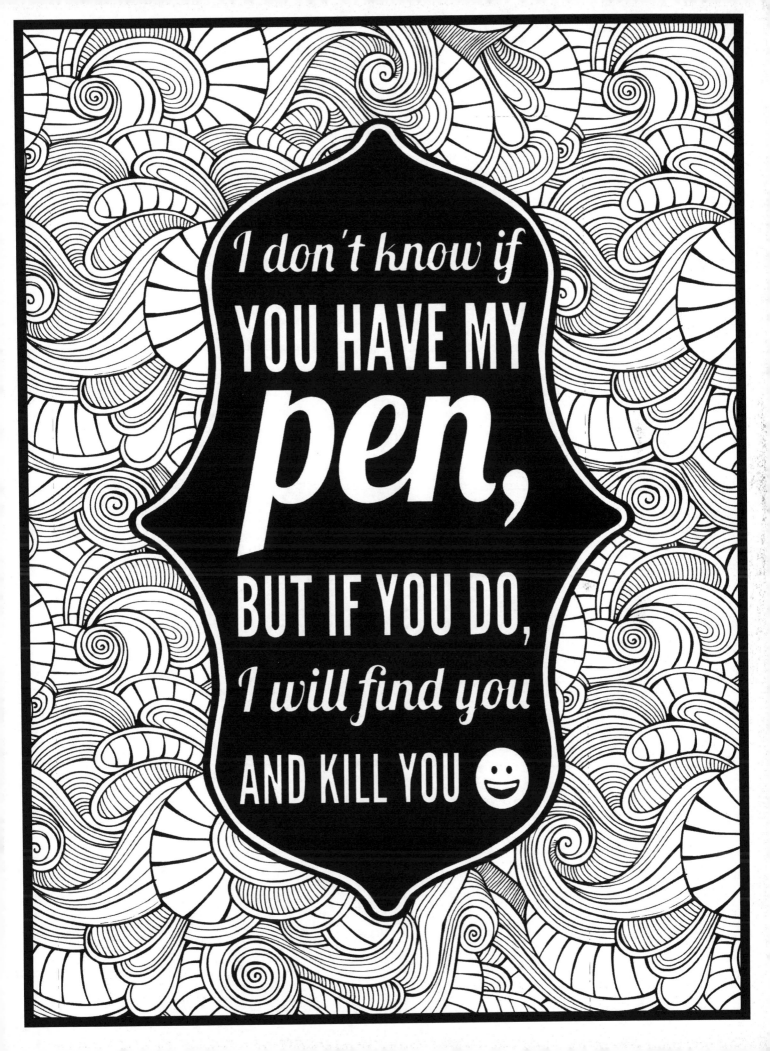

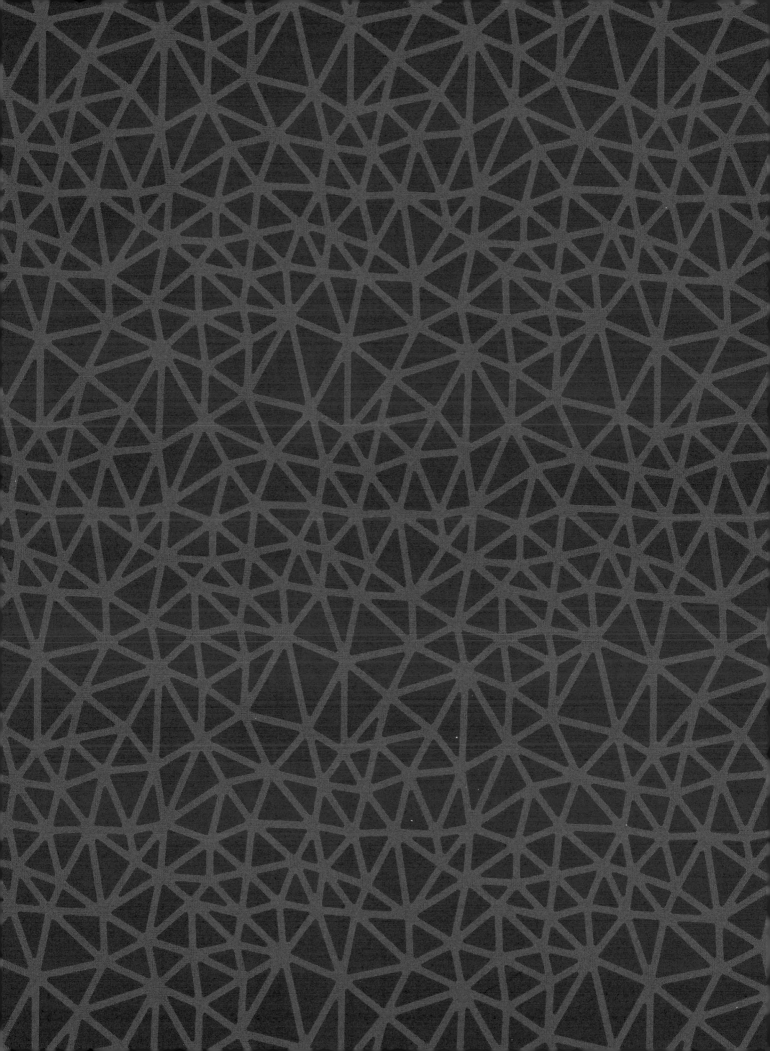

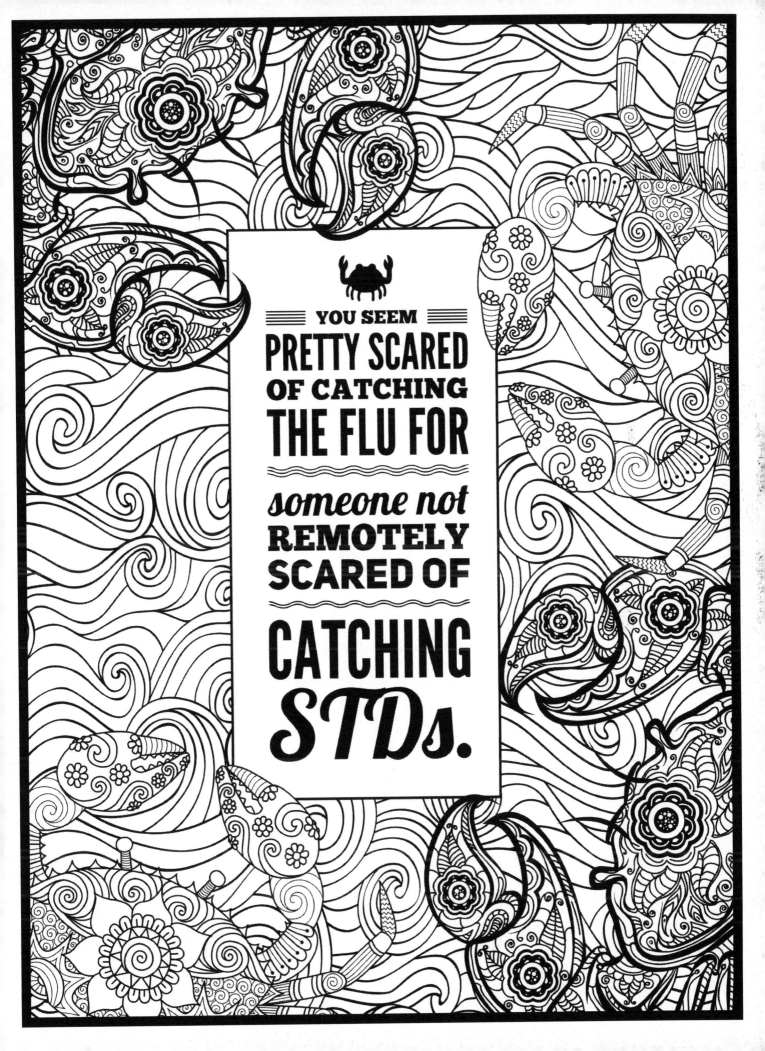

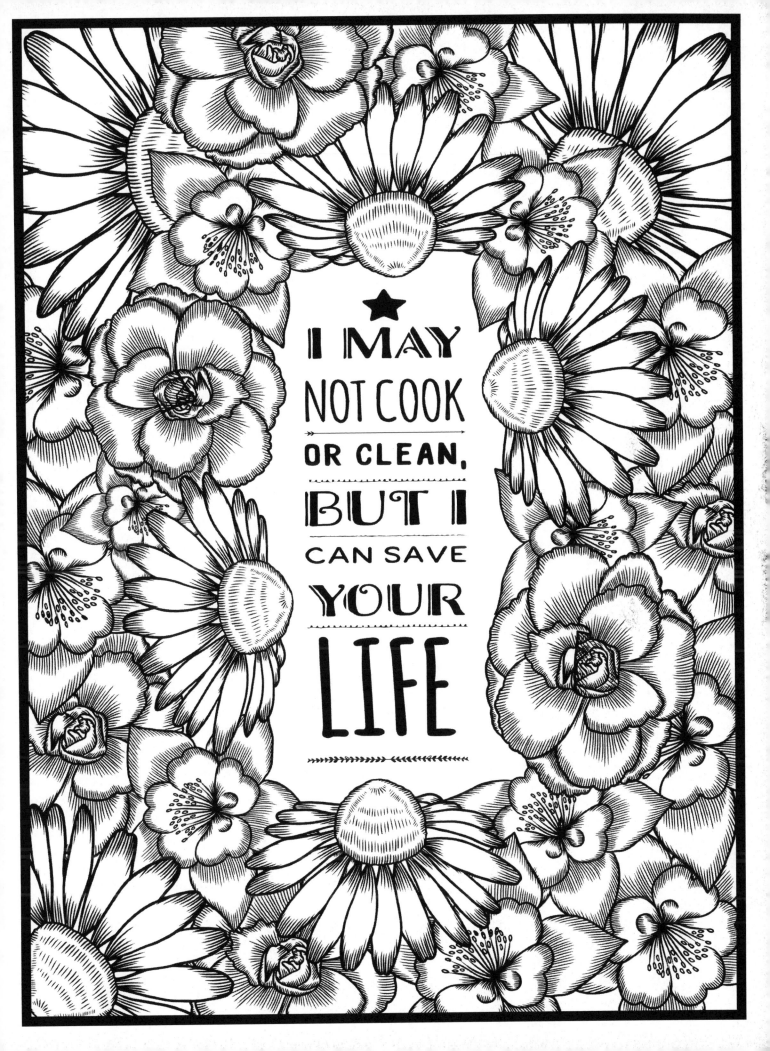

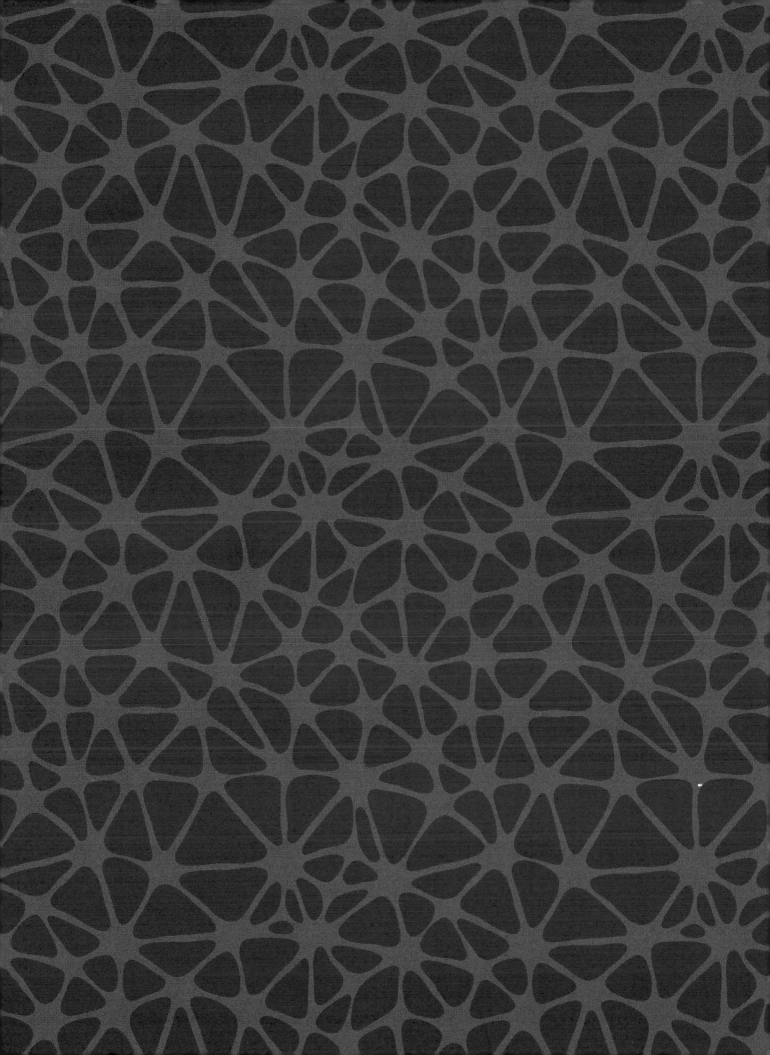

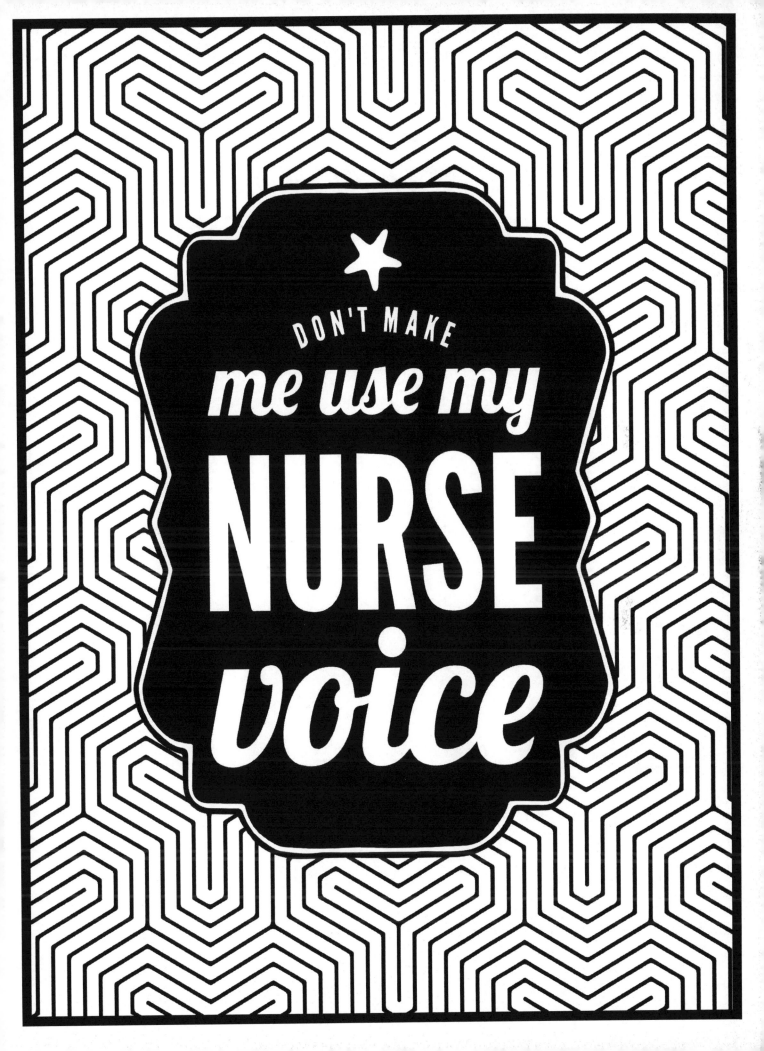

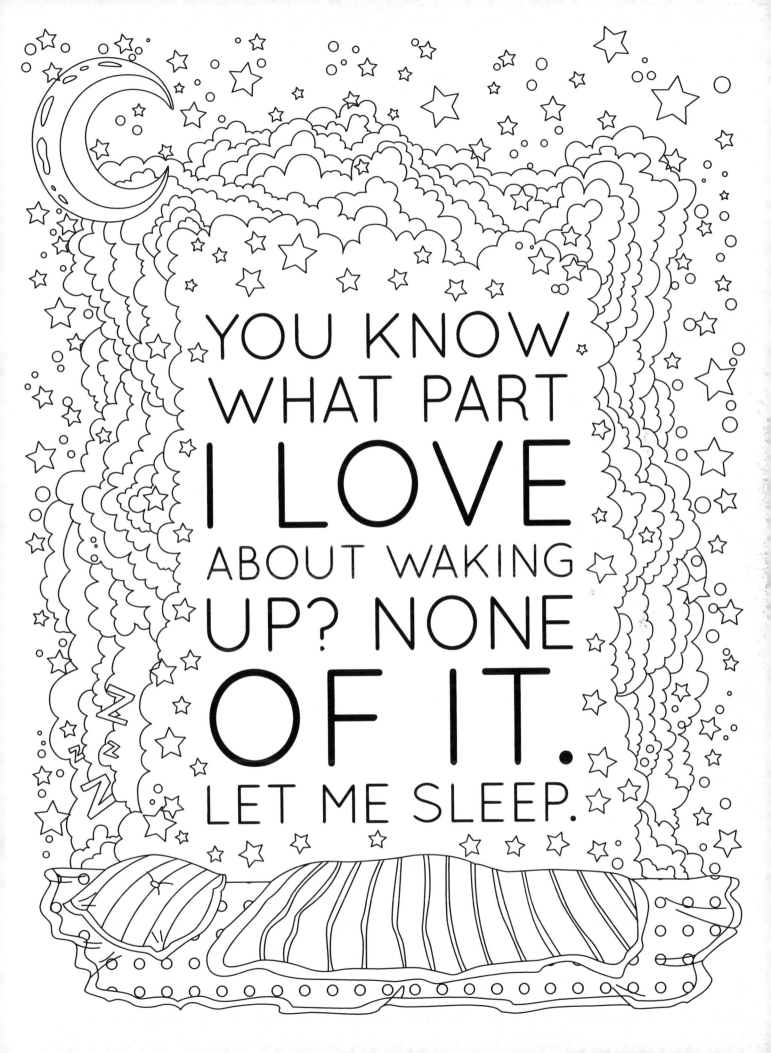

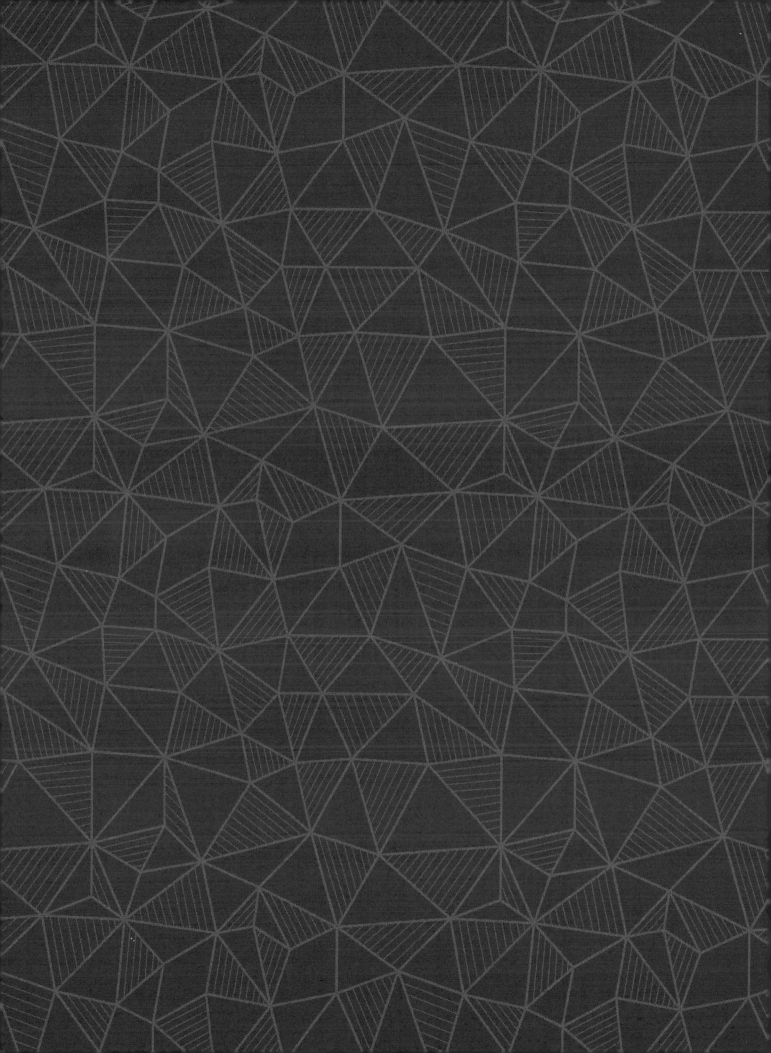

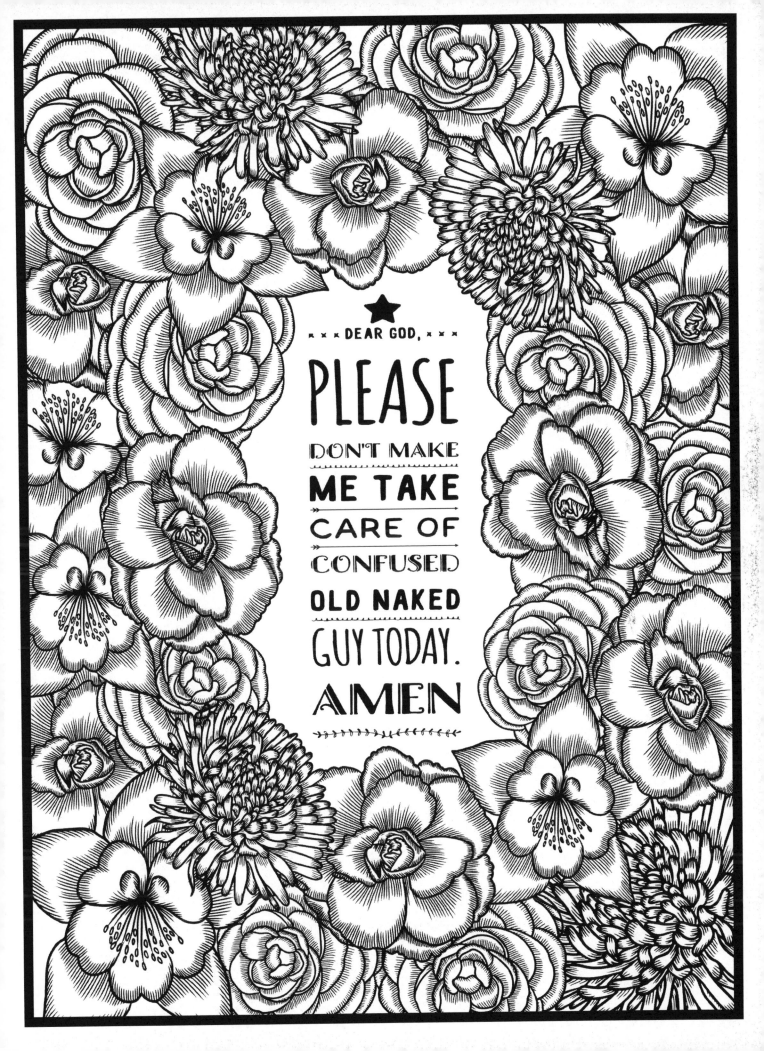

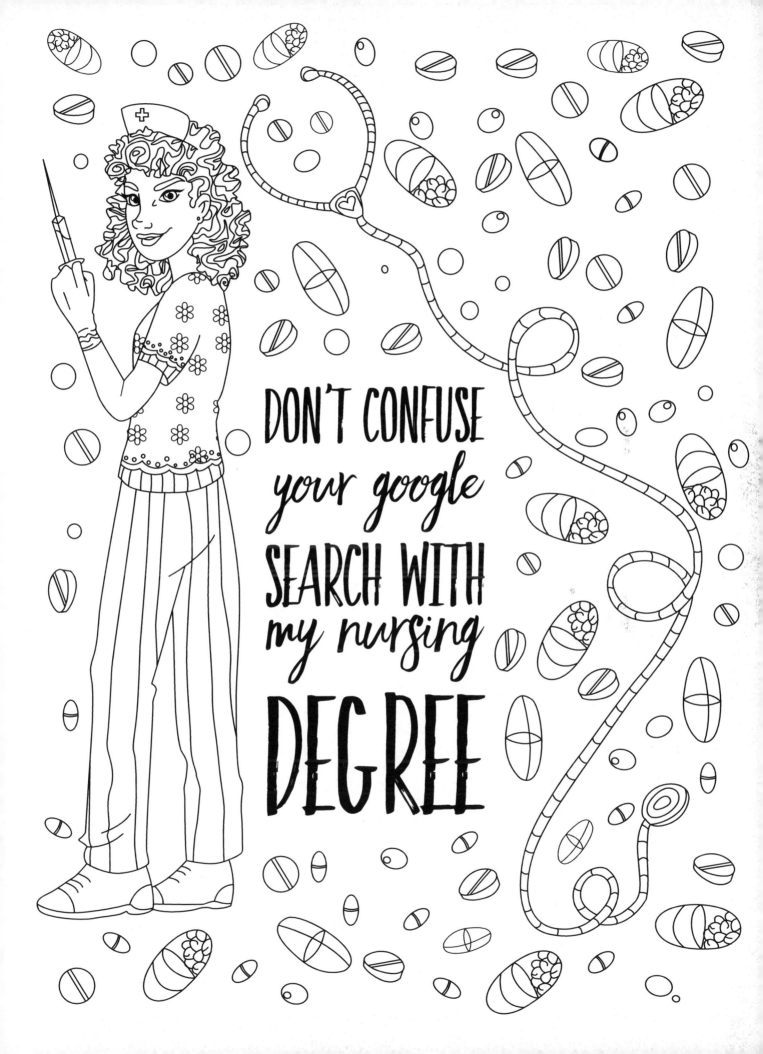

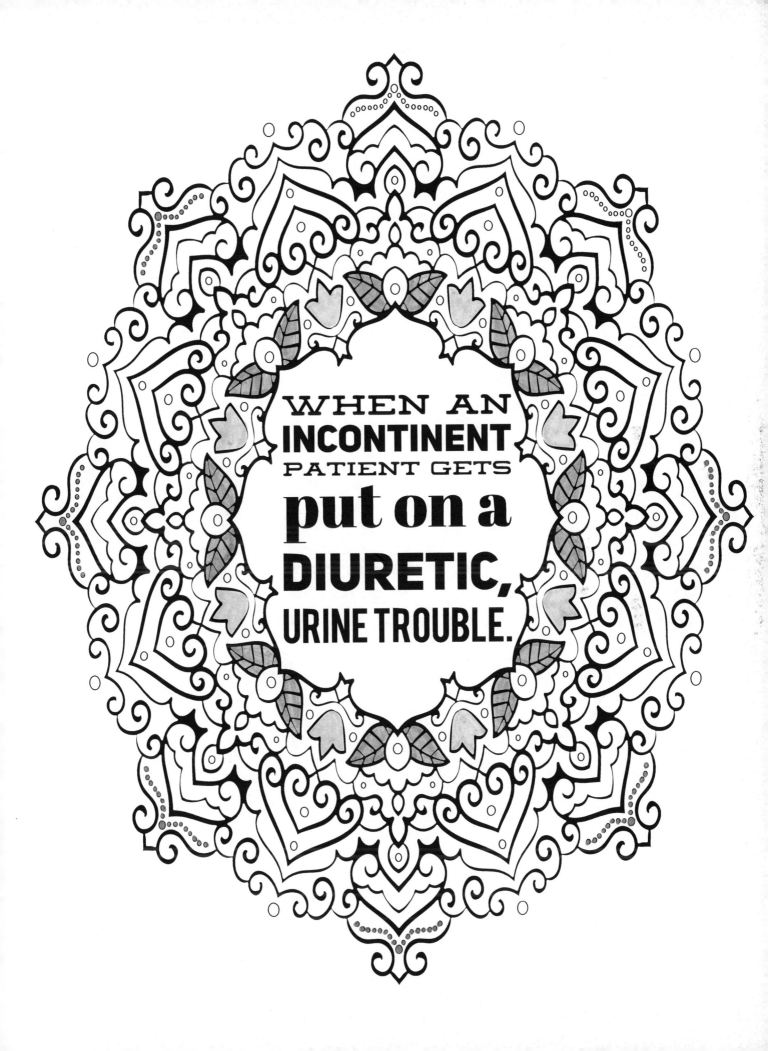

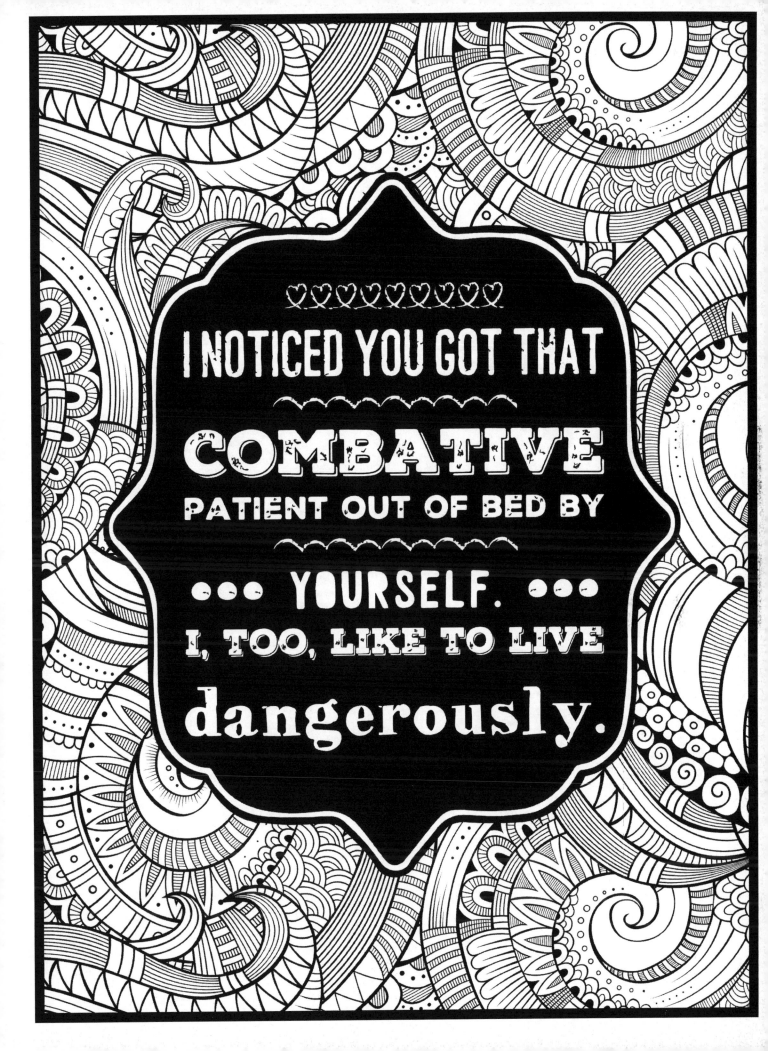

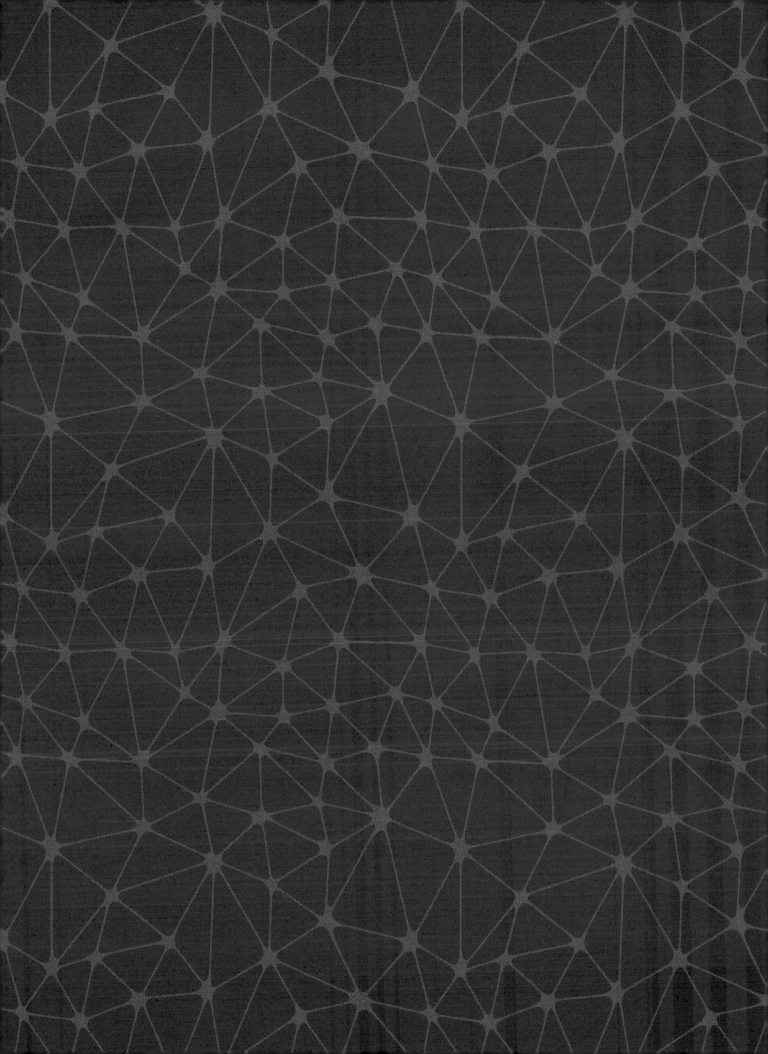

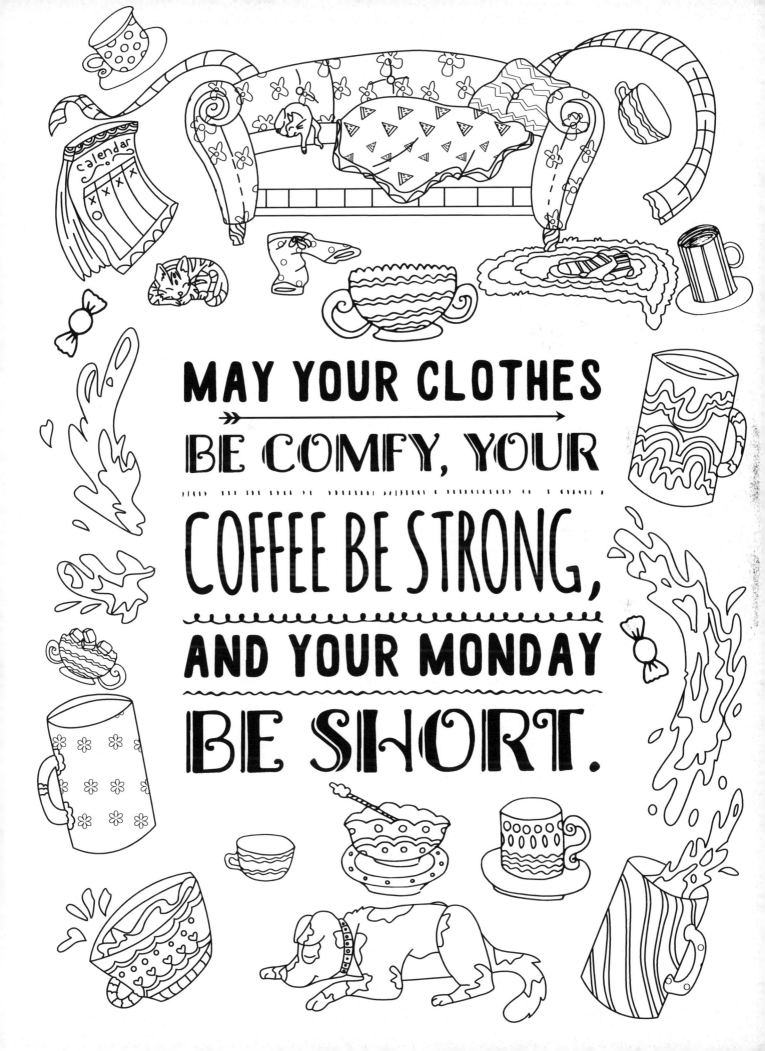

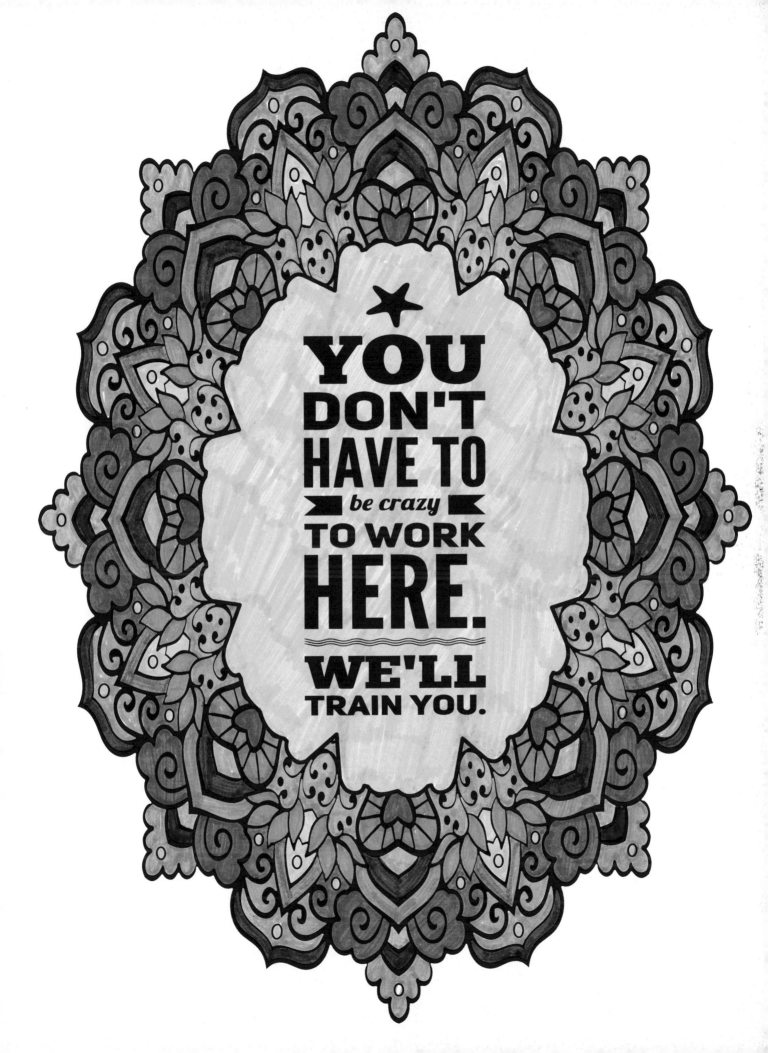

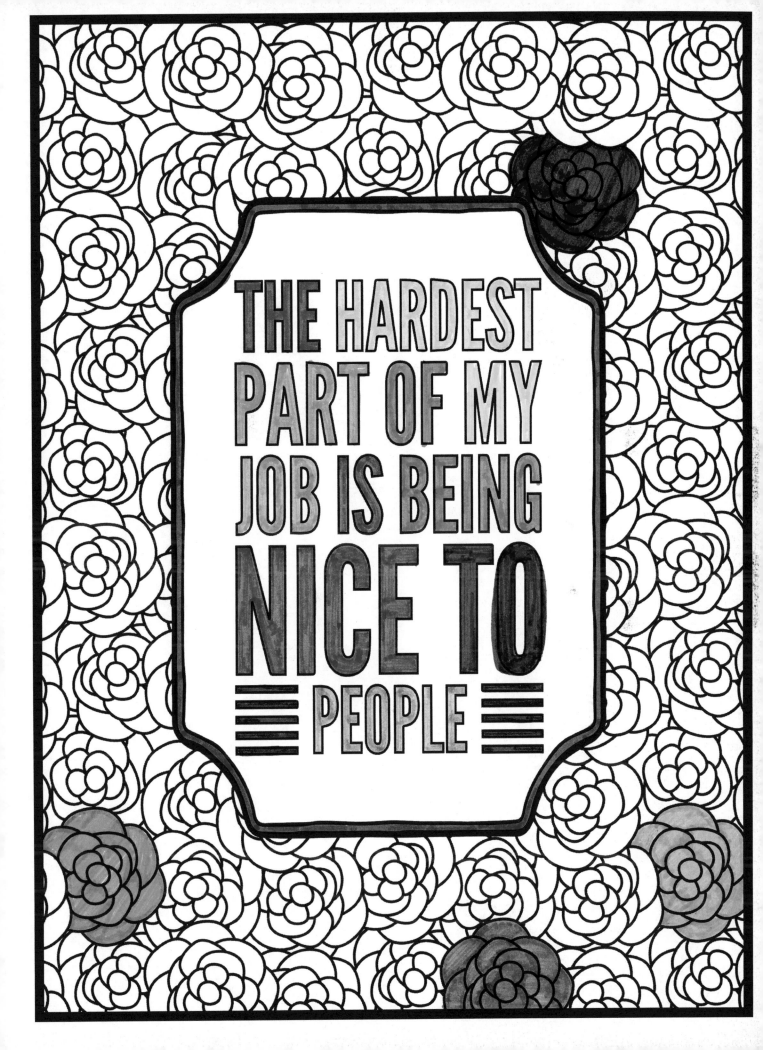

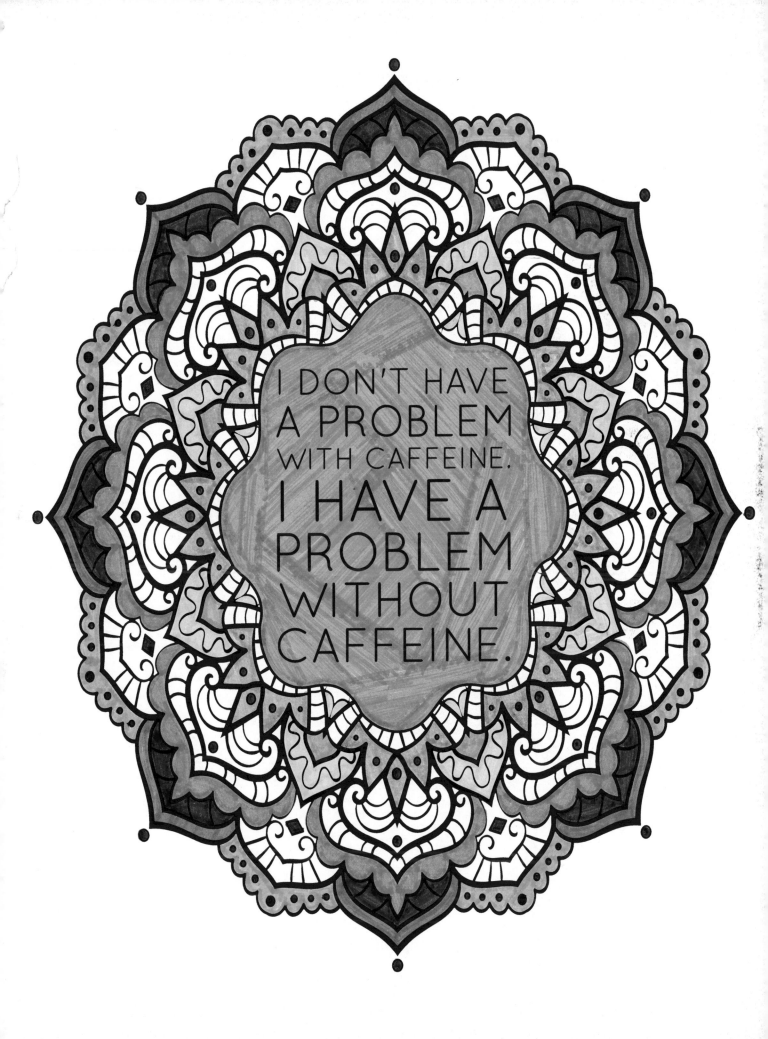

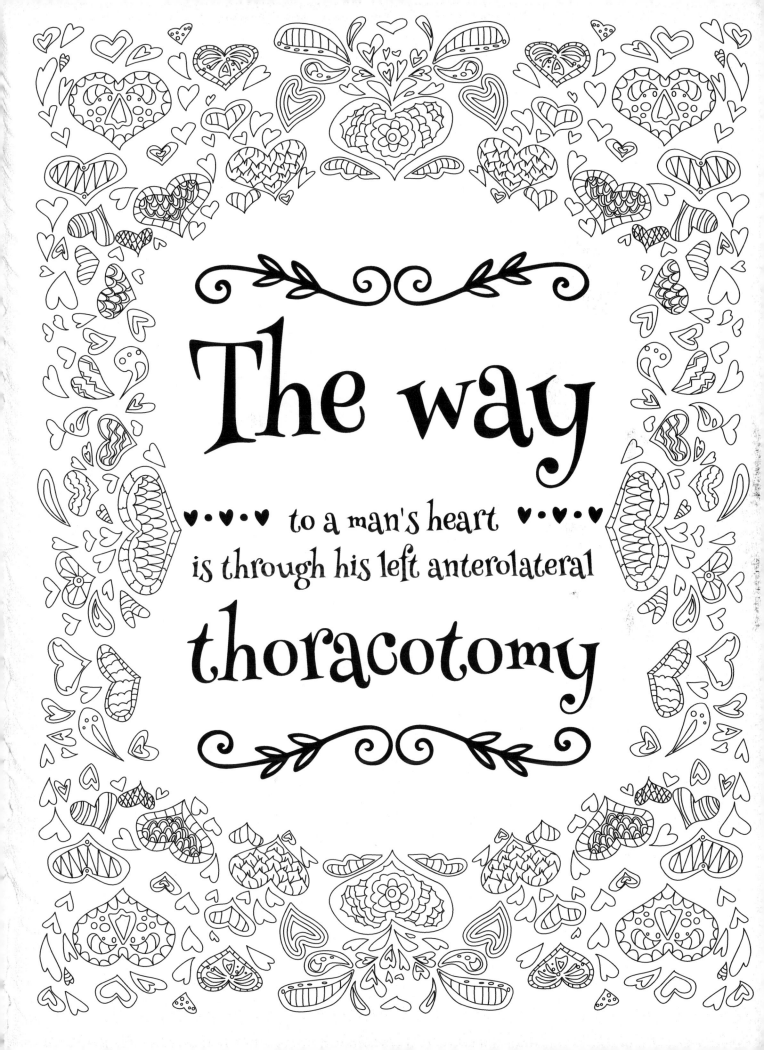

The way

•·•♥ to a man's heart ♥•·•♥
is through his left anterolateral

thoracotomy

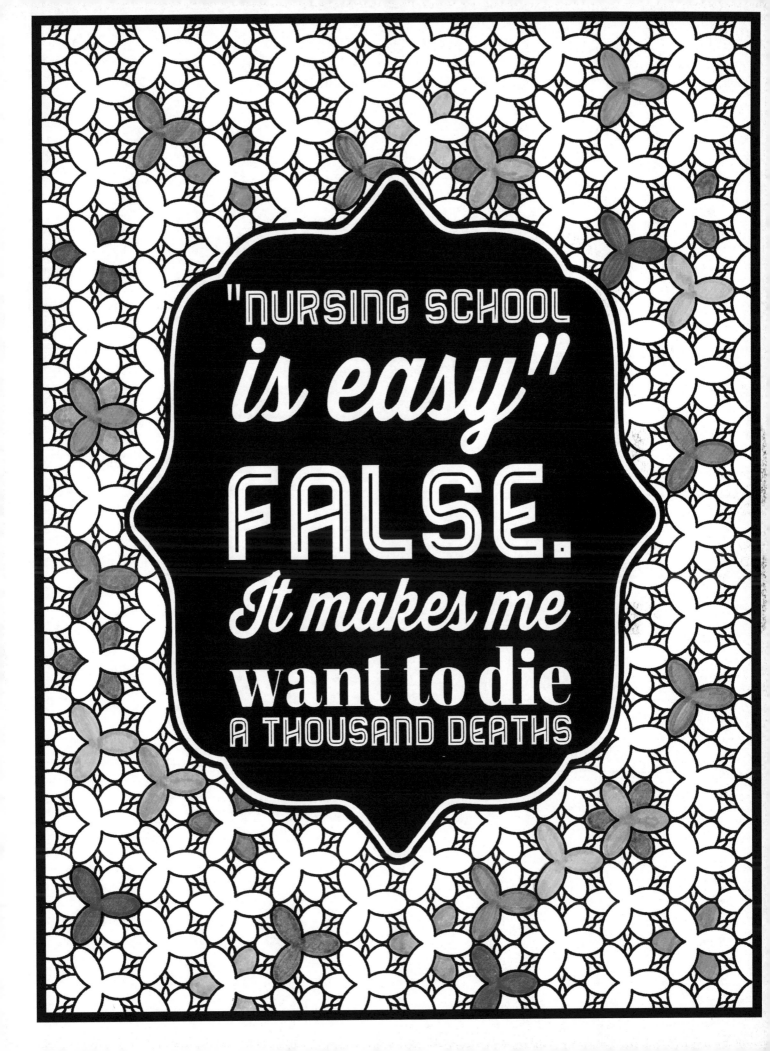

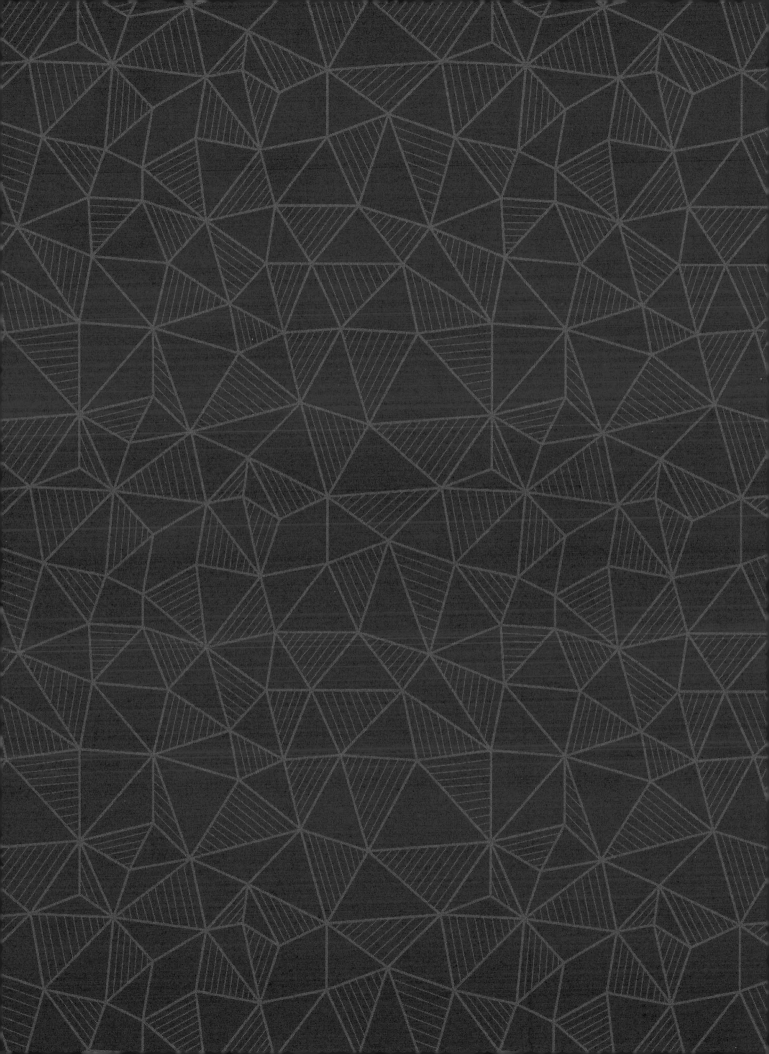

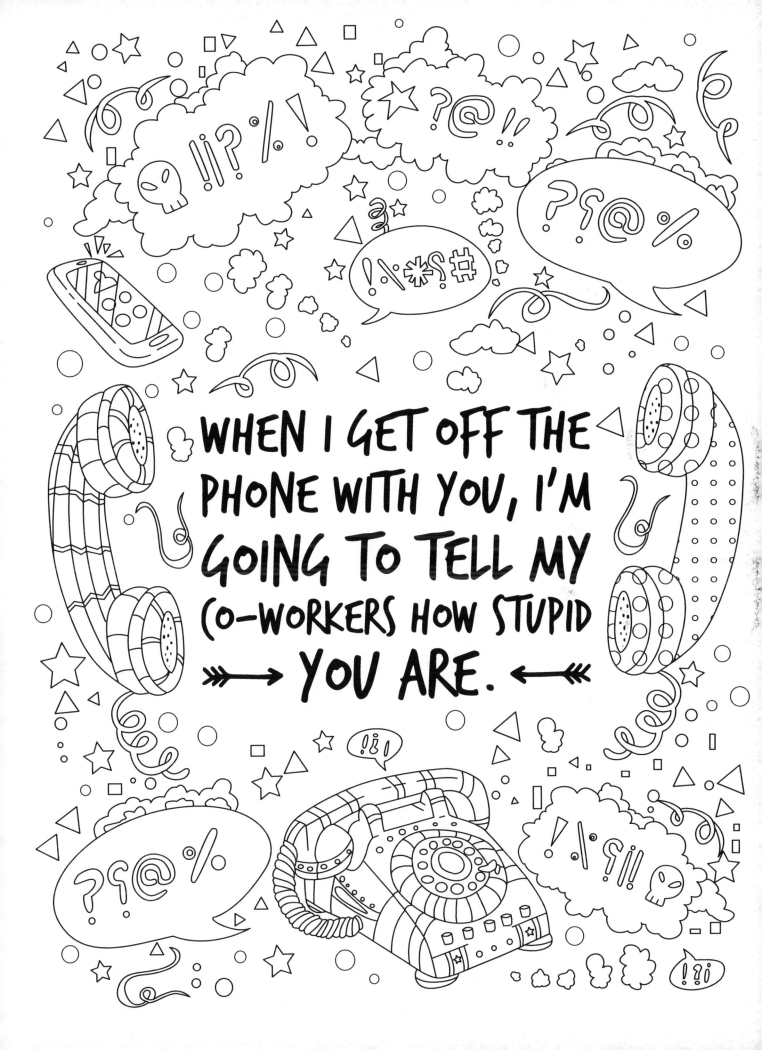

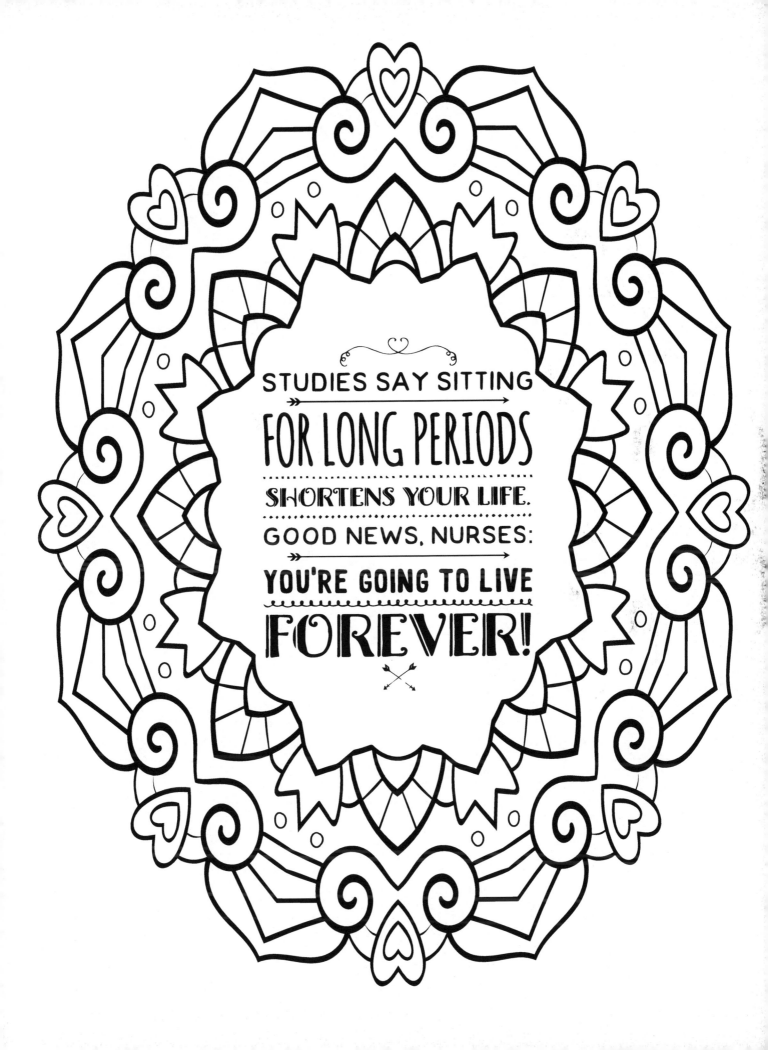

STUDIES SAY SITTING
FOR LONG PERIODS
SHORTENS YOUR LIFE.
GOOD NEWS, NURSES:
YOU'RE GOING TO LIVE
FOREVER!

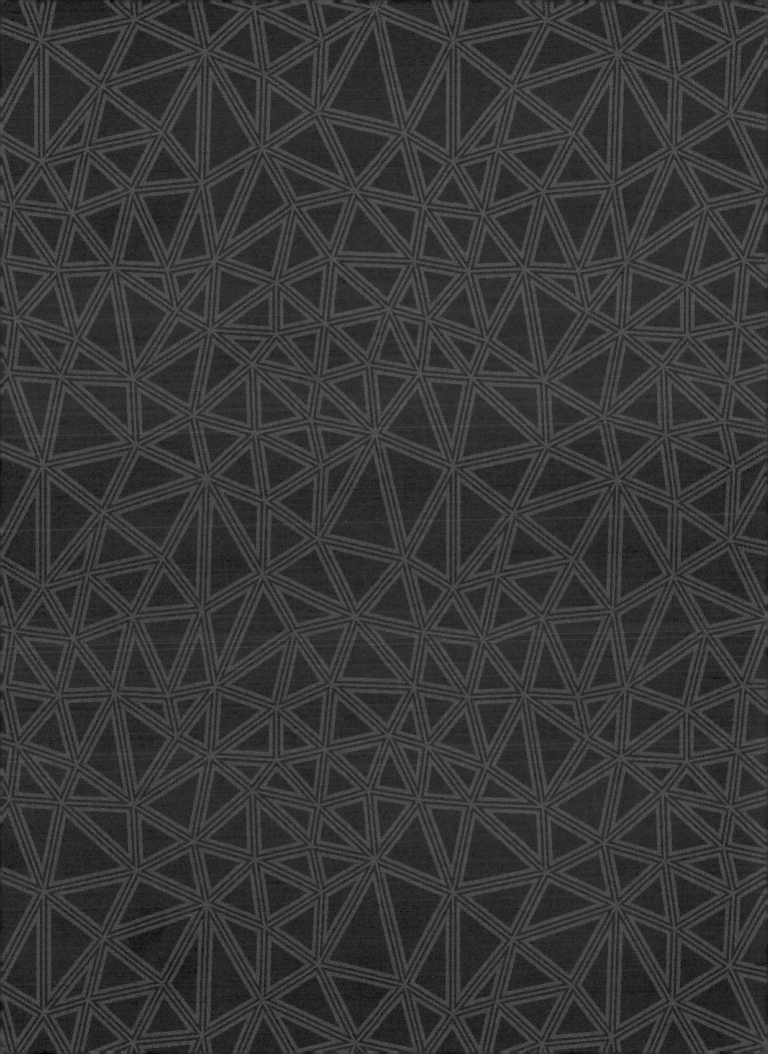

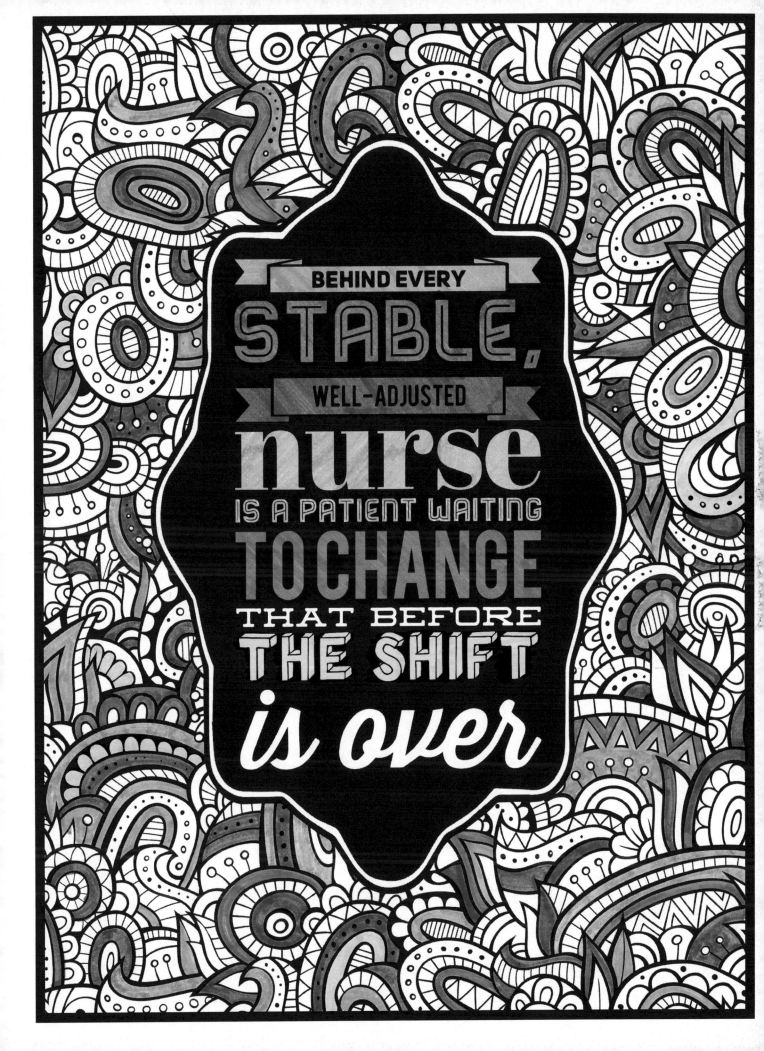

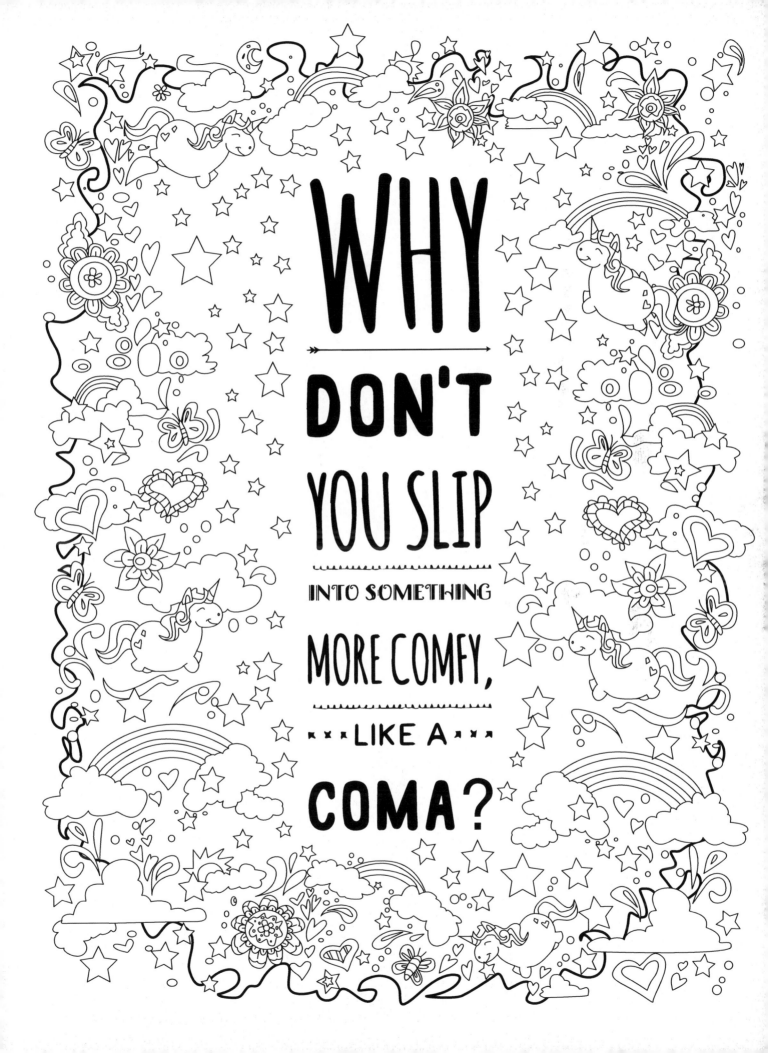

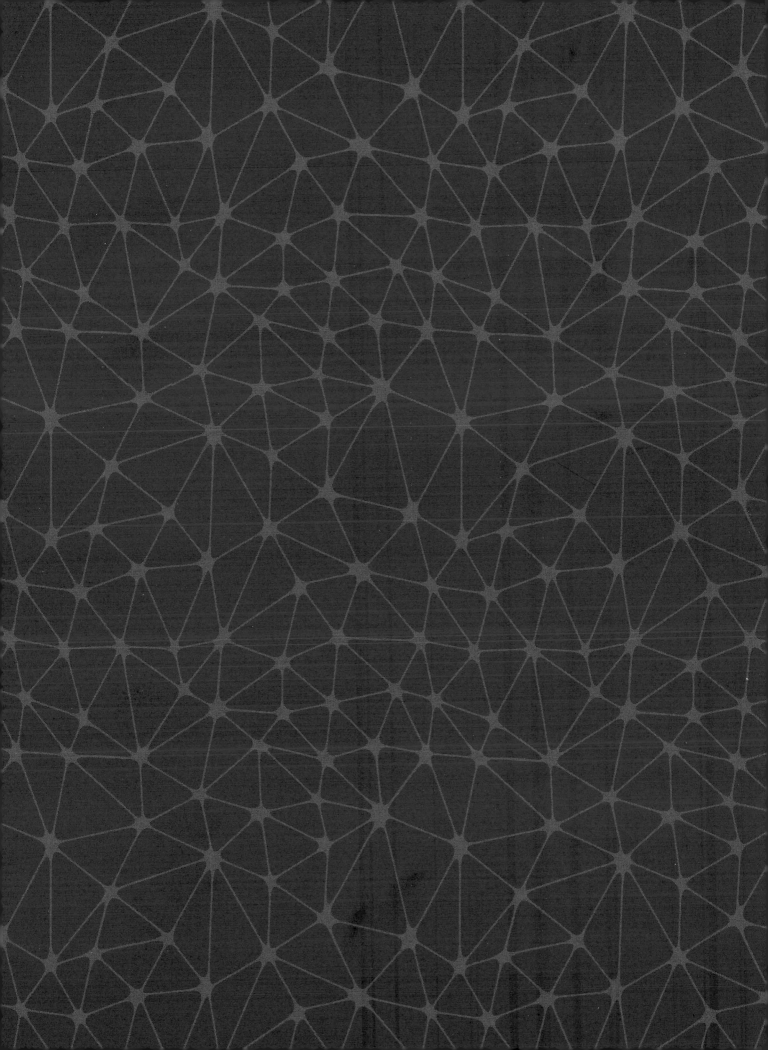